KEGEL EXERCISES FOR MEN

Daily Kegel Routine For Men With Practical And Easy-To-Follow Exercises To Integrate Into Your Busy Life For Maximum Benefits

CONTENT

INTRODUCTION

Erectile dysfunction (ED) is a condition that affects millions of men worldwide, often leading to physical and emotional challenges. While there are many potential causes and treatments, one often-overlooked yet highly effective solution lies in the strength of your pelvic floor muscles. These muscles play a crucial role in sexual function, bladder and bowel control, and overall vitality. Strengthening them can be transformative for your health and confidence.

This book, Kegel Exercise for Men: Strengthen Pelvic Floor Muscles for Overcoming Erectile Dysfunction and Boosting Sexual

Function for Optimum Health, is your comprehensive guide to unlocking the potential of your pelvic floor muscles. Through practical exercises and easy-to-follow routines, you'll learn how to take control of your health and achieve results that last a lifetime.

The Importance of Pelvic Floor Muscles:

Your pelvic floor muscles are a group of tissues that stretch like a hammock across the bottom of your pelvis, supporting vital organs such as the bladder, bowel, and, for men, the prostate. Despite their critical role, these muscles are often neglected until a problem arises.

Healthy pelvic floor muscles are essential for maintaining control over urination and bowel movements, preventing discomfort and inconvenience. More importantly, they are vital for robust sexual health. Weak pelvic floor muscles can lead to challenges such as erectile dysfunction, premature ejaculation, and reduced sexual stamina. Understanding their anatomy and importance is the first step in reclaiming control over your body.

Understanding Erectile Dysfunction (ED) and Its Causes:

Erectile dysfunction is not merely a symptom of aging; it's often a result of underlying factors that can be addressed. Common causes include stress, poor circulation, hormonal imbalances, and weak pelvic floor muscles.

Weak pelvic floor muscles can impair the ability to maintain erections by reducing blood flow to the penis and weakening the support necessary for optimal function. By targeting and strengthening these muscles, you can address one of the root causes of ED effectively and naturally.

Benefits of Kegel Exercises for Men:

Kegel exercises, designed specifically to strengthen the pelvic floor, offer a host of benefits:

1: Improved Erectile Function: Stronger pelvic floor muscles enhance blood flow and support for erections, leading to noticeable improvements in performance.

2: Enhanced Bladder and Bowel Control: Say goodbye to leaks and embarrassing accidents by improving your control and confidence.

3: Boosted Sexual Performance and Stamina: By building pelvic floor strength, you can experience heightened pleasure, greater endurance, and renewed energy in intimate moments.

How This Book Will Help You:

This guide is designed with you in mind, providing:

1: Practical, Easy-to-Follow Exercises: Step-by-step instructions and illustrations make it simple to master Kegel exercises, even if you're a beginner.

2: Realistic Daily Routines: Incorporate these exercises seamlessly into your busy life, with routines that take just minutes a day.

Whether your goal is to overcome ED, improve your overall health, or boost your confidence in the bedroom, this book will equip you with the tools and knowledge you need to succeed. By dedicating just a few minutes a day to strengthening your pelvic floor, you can unlock a new level of vitality, wellness, and satisfaction.

GETTING TO KNOW YOUR PELVIC FLOOR

Understanding your pelvic floor is essential to mastering Kegel exercises and unlocking their full potential for improved sexual health, urinary control, and overall well-being. This chapter delves into the anatomy of the male pelvic floor, signs of pelvic floor weakness, and how to assess your pelvic floor strength.

Anatomy of the Male Pelvic Floor:

The male pelvic floor is a complex network of muscles, ligaments, and connective tissues that play a vital role in sexual and urinary functions. Key muscles include:

Key Muscles Involved

1. Pubococcygeus (PC) Muscle: Often referred to as the "powerhouse" of the pelvic floor, the PC muscle stretches from the pubic bone to the tailbone. It provides support to the bladder and rectum and is instrumental in controlling urination and ejaculation.

2. Bulbocavernosus Muscle: This muscle surrounds the base of the penis and helps control the flow of urine. It also contributes to the force of ejaculation and plays a role in penile rigidity during erections.

3. Ischiocavernosus Muscle: Located along the sides of the penis, this muscle helps maintain an erection by restricting blood flow out of the penile tissues.

4. Levator Ani Group: A group of muscles, including the puborectalis and iliococcygeus, which supports the pelvic organs and helps with bowel movements and urinary control.

Functions of These Muscles:

1: Sexual Health: The pelvic floor muscles enhance blood flow to the penis, contributing to stronger erections and more controlled ejaculations.

2: Urinary Control: These muscles ensure proper functioning of the bladder and sphincters, preventing issues like incontinence.

3: Supportive Role: By supporting the pelvic organs, these muscles maintain proper alignment and function of the bladder, prostate, and rectum.

Signs of a Weak Pelvic Floor:

Recognizing the signs of pelvic floor weakness is the first step toward addressing the issue. Weak pelvic floor muscles can lead to a range of symptoms that may interfere with daily life.

Symptoms to Watch Out For:

I. Urinary Leakage: Difficulty controlling urine flow, especially during sneezing, coughing, or lifting heavy objects.

II. Erectile Dysfunction (ED): Difficulty achieving or maintaining an erection due to reduced blood flow and muscle support.

III. Premature Ejaculation: Challenges in controlling ejaculation.

IV. Frequent Urination: An increased urge to urinate, even when the bladder isn't full.

Link between Pelvic Floor Weakness and ED:

Pelvic floor dysfunction can contribute to ED by reducing

blood flow and weakening the structural support needed for an erection. Studies have shown that targeted pelvic floor exercises, such as Kegels, can significantly improve erectile function by strengthening these critical muscles.

Assessing Your Pelvic Floor Strength:

Before beginning Kegel exercises, it's important to assess the current strength of your pelvic floor muscles. This self-awareness will help tailor your exercise routine to your specific needs.

Self-Assessment Techniques:

1. The Stop-Test: While urinating, attempt to stop the flow of urine midstream. If you can do so effectively, your pelvic floor muscles are likely functioning well. If not, this may indicate weakness.

2. Erection Test: Observe the firmness and angle of your erections. Reduced rigidity may point to pelvic floor weakness.

3. Palpation: Gently press on the area between your scrotum and anus (perineum) while contracting your pelvic muscles. A firm response indicates muscle engagement.

When to Consult a Professional:

I. Persistent Symptoms: If you experience ongoing urinary leakage, ED, or pelvic pain, consulting a healthcare professional is advisable.

II. Uncertainty about Technique: If you're unsure about locating or engaging your pelvic floor muscles, a physiotherapist specializing in pelvic health can provide guidance.

III. Rehabilitation Needs: For individuals recovering from surgery or injuries affecting the pelvic area, professional advice can ensure safe and effective exercise.

UNDERSTANDING KEGEL EXERCISES

What Are Kegel Exercises?

Kegel exercises, named after Dr. Arnold Kegel, are simple yet powerful movements designed to strengthen the pelvic floor muscles. These muscles, located at the base of the pelvis, play a crucial role in supporting the bladder, rectum, and, in men, the prostate and urethra. Originally developed in the 1940s for women dealing with urinary incontinence post-childbirth, Kegel exercises have since been recognized as highly beneficial for men as well.

Origins and Purpose:

The concept of Kegel exercises stems from the understanding that strengthening internal muscles can significantly improve bodily control and function. For men, these exercises are primarily aimed at:

I. Enhancing bladder and bowel control

II. Supporting prostate health

III. Improving sexual function by addressing erectile dysfunction (ED) and enhancing performance

Despite their clinical origins, Kegels are now widely recommended as a natural and non-invasive way to address various health concerns and improve quality of life.

Myths and Misconceptions:

Kegel exercises are often misunderstood, leading to hesitation or improper practice. Common myths include:

I. Only for women: While initially targeted at women, Kegels are just as effective for men, addressing issues like ED, incontinence, and post-surgery recovery.

II. Immediate results: While beneficial, Kegels require consistent practice over weeks or months to yield noticeable improvements.

III. Difficult to perform: Kegels are deceptively simple and can be done almost anywhere without special equipment.

By debunking these misconceptions, more men can embrace the potential of Kegel exercises to enhance their health and confidence.

How Kegel Exercises Work:

Kegel exercises specifically target the pelvic floor muscles, which are often overlooked in traditional fitness routines. Strengthening these muscles can have profound effects on overall well-being.

Targeting the Right Muscles:

Identifying the pelvic floor muscles is the first step in practicing Kegels effectively. These muscles can be located by stopping the flow of urine midstream or tightening as if trying to prevent gas from passing. Once identified, these muscles are isolated and engaged during Kegel exercises.

Mechanisms Behind Improved Sexual Function and ED Relief:

The pelvic floor muscles play a pivotal role in sexual health. By strengthening them, men may experience:

I. Improved blood flow: Stronger pelvic muscles enhance circulation to the genital area, supporting erections.

II. Better control: Increased muscle strength can lead to improved stamina and control during intimacy.

III. Support for ED treatment: For men with erectile dysfunction,

Kegels can complement medical treatments by addressing underlying muscle weakness or circulation issues.

These mechanisms make Kegels a valuable tool in promoting both physical and sexual health.

Who Can Benefit from Kegel Exercises?

Kegel exercises offer benefits for men of all ages and can be tailored to address specific health conditions or concerns.

Men of All Ages:

From young men seeking to enhance performance to older individuals aiming to maintain pelvic health, Kegels are universally beneficial. Regular practice can:

I. Prevent potential issues related to aging

II. Enhance confidence and well-being

Specific Conditions:

Kegels are particularly advantageous for men dealing with:

I. Erectile Dysfunction (ED): By strengthening pelvic muscles, men can experience better blood flow and improved erectile function.

II. Incontinence: For those struggling with bladder or bowel control, Kegels can help regain mastery over these functions.

III.   Post-Prostate   Surgery Recovery: After prostate surgery, the pelvic floor muscles may weaken. Kegels can expedite recovery, restoring control and function.

By understanding the wide-ranging benefits of Kegel exercises, men can adopt this practice as a vital component of their health regimen.

EASY KEGEL EXERCISES FOR BEGINNERS

Kegel exercises are an effective way for men to strengthen their pelvic floor muscles, leading to improved urinary control, sexual health, and overall well-being. This chapter will guide you through simple exercises designed for beginners, ensuring you start on the right path to success.

Identifying the Right Muscles:

Before starting Kegel exercises, it is crucial to locate and engage the correct muscles. The pelvic floor muscles support the bladder and bowel, playing a key role in urinary and sexual function.

Techniques to Locate the Pelvic Floor Muscles:

I. Stopping the Flow of Urine: The easiest way to identify your pelvic floor muscles is to attempt stopping your urine midstream. The muscles you engage to achieve this are your pelvic floor muscles. Note: This is only a diagnostic technique and should not be done regularly to avoid disrupting normal bladder function.

II. Checking with a Mirror: Sit or lie down with a mirror positioned to view your perineum (the area between your anus and scrotum). Contract the muscles as if trying to stop passing gas; the area will visibly lift or tighten.

III. Finger Test: Insert a clean finger into your rectum and tighten the muscles as though holding in gas. You should feel a tightening around your finger.

Tips to Avoid Engaging the Wrong Muscles:

I. Avoid tensing your buttocks, thighs, or abdomen during the exercise.

II. Keep your breathing relaxed to ensure you're not holding your breath.

III. Practice in a quiet and comfortable space where you can focus fully on the correct muscle engagement.

Basic Kegel Exercise Techniques:

Once you have identified the correct muscles, you can begin with simple Kegel exercises. These techniques are foundational for building strength and control in your pelvic floor.

Slow Contractions:

1. Engage the Muscles: Slowly tighten your pelvic floor muscles, as if trying to stop urine flow.

2. Hold the Contraction: Maintain the squeeze for 3-5 seconds. Gradually increase this to 10 seconds as you gain strength.

3. Relax: Release the muscles fully and rest for 5 seconds before repeating.

4. Repetitions: Aim for 10 repetitions per session, and try to complete three sessions per day.

Quick Flicks:

1. Contract Quickly: Tighten your pelvic floor muscles as quickly and firmly as possible.

2. Release Immediately: Let go of the contraction without holding it.

3. Repetitions: Perform 10 quick flicks in a row. This exercise helps improve the responsiveness of the pelvic floor muscles.

Relaxation and Release:

1. Consciously Relax: Focus on fully relaxing your pelvic floor muscles between contractions. This prevents tension and promotes better recovery.

2. Deep Breathing: Combine with slow, deep breaths to ensure

you're not inadvertently tensing other muscles.

3. Practice Duration: Spend 2-3 minutes focusing solely on relaxation after completing other Kegel exercises.

Common Mistakes to Avoid:

While Kegel exercises are simple, improper practice can reduce their effectiveness or even cause discomfort. Avoid these common pitfalls:

Overworking the Muscles:

I. Rest Periods: Overdoing Kegel exercises can lead to muscle fatigue and strain. Ensure you're giving your pelvic floor muscles time to recover.

II. Gradual Progression: Start with manageable repetitions and increase only as your strength improves.

Holding Your Breath:

I. Stay Relaxed: Many beginners unintentionally hold their breath while contracting the muscles. Focus on steady, rhythmic breathing to keep your body relaxed.

Engaging the Wrong Muscles:

I. Target Accuracy: Tensing your buttocks, thighs, or abdomen can negate the benefits of Kegel exercises. Regularly check to ensure you're engaging only the pelvic floor muscles.

By following these beginner-friendly techniques and tips, you can effectively strengthen your pelvic floor muscles without strain or frustration. With consistency and proper form, you'll soon experience the benefits of improved control and confidence.

ADVANCED KEGEL WORKOUT ROUTINE

Kegel exercises are a foundational practice for improving pelvic floor strength and enhancing overall well-being. As with any fitness regimen, progression is key to unlocking greater benefits. This chapter focuses on advanced techniques to elevate your Kegel workout routine.

Progressing Your Routine:

Increasing Repetitions and Duration:

As you grow more comfortable with your initial Kegel exercises, it's important to gradually increase both the number of repetitions and the duration of each contraction. Here's how:

I. Repetitions: Begin by adding a few extra repetitions each week. For instance, if you started with 10 contractions per session, aim to reach 15 to 20 over time.

II. Duration: Extend the time of each contraction. If you're holding for 3 seconds, try increasing to 5 or 10 seconds as your endurance improves.

III. Frequency: Perform your exercises more frequently, progressing from once daily to two or three sessions per day.

Consistency in these adjustments ensures steady improvement

without overstraining your muscles.

Adding Variations to Exercises:

Introducing variety keeps your routine engaging and targets different aspects of pelvic floor strength. Consider these variations:

I. Quick Contractions: Alternate between quick pulses and longer holds to challenge muscle responsiveness.

II. Alternating Positions: Practice Kegels in different body positions, such as lying down, sitting, standing, or even on all fours.

III. Reverse Kegels: Focus on gently pushing out or relaxing the pelvic floor muscles, complementing the contraction phase.

These variations help maintain balance and flexibility in your pelvic floor muscles.

Incorporating Resistance and Weights:

For those seeking a greater challenge, resistance training can amplify the effectiveness of Kegel exercises.

Using Tools Like Kegel Weights (Optional)

Kegel weights are designed to add resistance, making your pelvic floor muscles work harder. To integrate them:

1. Choose the Right Weight: Start with a lightweight option and gradually increase as you gain strength.

2. Proper Insertion: Follow the manufacturer's instructions to safely and comfortably position the weight.

3. Perform Kegels: Focus on holding the weight in place during contractions.

4. Progress Gradually: As with any exercise, increase the weight or duration over time.

Safety Precautions:

I. Always consult a healthcare professional before incorporating weights.

II. Avoid using weights if you experience pain or discomfort.

III. Practice proper hygiene to prevent infections.

IV. Do not overuse weights; limit sessions to avoid muscle fatigue.

Integrating Kegel Exercises with Full-Body Workouts:

Combining Kegels with other exercises can amplify results and build synergy between your core and pelvic floor.

Core and Pelvic Floor Synergy:

The pelvic floor is a key component of your core. Strengthening this connection can improve posture, stability, and overall strength. Focus on engaging your pelvic floor muscles during core workouts like planks or leg raises.

Exercises Like Squats and Bridges:

These full-body movements naturally engage the pelvic floor, making them ideal for integration:

I. Squats: As you lower into a squat, consciously contract your pelvic floor. Release the contraction as you return to standing.

II. Bridges: While lifting your hips in a bridge pose, engage your pelvic floor. Hold briefly at the top before lowering down.

III. Deadlifts: Maintain pelvic floor engagement throughout the lifting motion to support your lower back and enhance muscle activation.

By progressively enhancing your Kegel routine, integrating resistance tools, and combining exercises with full-body movements, you can achieve advanced pelvic floor strength and overall well-being. Remember, consistency and mindful practice are the foundations of success in any workout regimen.

DAILY KEGEL EXERCISE PLAN

Kegel exercises can significantly improve pelvic floor strength and overall health when practiced consistently. This chapter provides a structured approach to integrating Kegel exercises into your daily routine, offering practical tips and a sample plan tailored to different levels of experience.

Building a Consistent Routine:

Consistency is the key to reaping the benefits of Kegel exercises. Incorporating these exercises into your daily schedule ensures that they become a natural part of your lifestyle. Here's how to create a balanced routine:

Morning, Afternoon, and Evening Exercises:

I. Morning: Start your day with a quick session to activate your pelvic floor muscles. Perform 5-10 repetitions of Kegel contractions before or after your morning routine, such as brushing your teeth or showering.

II. Afternoon: Take a short break during lunch or work to perform another set. Aim for 10-15 repetitions while seated or standing.

III. Evening: Wind down with a focused session before bedtime. Perform 15-20 repetitions to relax and strengthen your muscles before sleep.

Suggested Repetitions and Sets:

I. Beginners: Start with 1-2 sets of 5-10 repetitions per session. Focus on proper technique and avoid overexertion.

II. Intermediate: Gradually increase to 2-3 sets of 10-15 repetitions per session as your strength improves.

III. Advanced: Aim for 3-4 sets of 15-20 repetitions, incorporating longer holds and quicker contractions.

Tips for Sticking to Your Routine:

Establishing a habit can be challenging, but these strategies can help you stay consistent:

Setting Reminders:

I. Use smartphone alarms or apps to schedule reminders for your Kegel exercises.

II. Place sticky notes in visible locations, such as your bathroom mirror or desk.

Making It a Habit during Daily Activities:

I. Integrate Kegel exercises into routine tasks like commuting, waiting in line, or watching TV.

II. Pair Kegels with activities you do daily, such as checking emails or cooking dinner.

Sample Daily Kegel Exercise Plan:

This sample plan provides guidance for beginners, intermediates, and advanced practitioners. Adjust the plan as needed based on your comfort level and progress.

Beginner Level:

I. Morning: 1 set of 5 slow contractions (hold for 3 seconds each, then relax for 3 seconds).

II. Afternoon: 1 set of 5 quick contractions (squeeze and release rapidly).

III. Evening: 1 set of 5 slow contractions (hold for 3 seconds each, then relax for 3 seconds).

Intermediate Level:

I. Morning: 2 sets of 10 slow contractions (hold for 5 seconds each, and then relax for 5 seconds).

II. Afternoon: 1 set of 10 quick contractions, followed by 5 slow contractions.

III. Evening: 2 sets of 10 slow contractions (hold for 5 seconds each, and then relax for 5 seconds).

Advanced Level:

I. Morning: 3 sets of 15 slow contractions (hold for 10 seconds each, then relax for 10 seconds).

II. Afternoon: 2 sets of 15 quick contractions, followed by 10 slow contractions.

III. Evening: 3 sets of 15 slow contractions (hold for 10 seconds each, and then relax for 10 seconds).

By following this structured plan and incorporating the tips provided, you can build a consistent and effective Kegel exercise routine that strengthens your pelvic floor over time.

OVERCOMING ERECTILE DYSFUNCTION WITH KEGELS

Kegel exercises are a powerful tool in the fight against erectile dysfunction (ED). By strengthening the pelvic floor muscles, these exercises can enhance blood flow, improve control, and ultimately restore confidence and performance. This chapter explores the connection between Kegel exercises and ED, offers insights into combining them with other therapies, and provides tips for tracking progress effectively.

How Kegel Exercises Help with ED:

Scientific Evidence and Studies:

Research shows that pelvic floor muscle training can significantly improve erectile function. Studies have demonstrated that men who consistently perform Kegel exercises experience better blood flow to the penis, leading to stronger and more sustainable erections. One notable study published in the British Journal of Urology found that 40% of participants with ED regained normal erectile function after a dedicated regimen of pelvic floor exercises, while an additional 35% reported significant improvement.

These exercises target the bulbocavernosus muscle, which plays a crucial role in maintaining erections. Strengthening this muscle enhances its ability to compress veins and keep blood trapped in the penis, which is essential for achieving and maintaining firmness.

Real-Life Success Stories:

Many men have shared inspiring stories about overcoming ED through Kegel exercises. For example, John, a 45-year-old teacher, struggled with performance issues for years before discovering pelvic floor training. After committing to a daily routine, he noticed improvements within six weeks. Similarly, Michael, a 50-year-old businessman, combined Kegels with dietary changes and saw dramatic improvements in both his physical health and intimate life.

These stories highlight the transformative potential of Kegel exercises, particularly when integrated into a holistic approach to health.

Combining Kegel Exercises with Other Therapies:

Lifestyle Changes (Diet, Stress Management)

While Kegel exercises are effective on their own, combining them with lifestyle changes can accelerate results. A balanced diet rich in fruits, vegetables, lean proteins, and whole grains supports cardiovascular health, which is directly linked to erectile function. Avoiding processed foods and reducing alcohol intake can further enhance the benefits.

Stress management is equally important. Chronic stress increases cortisol levels, which can negatively impact testosterone and overall sexual health. Techniques such as mindfulness meditation, yoga, or even regular physical exercise can help reduce stress and complement the effects of Kegels.

Medications or Counseling When Necessary:

In some cases, ED may have psychological components, such as anxiety or depression, that Kegels alone cannot address. Counseling or therapy can help men identify and manage underlying emotional challenges. Medications like sildenafil (Viagra) or tadalafil (Cialis) may also provide temporary relief, allowing individuals to regain confidence while working on long-term solutions through exercises and lifestyle changes.

Combining these therapies with Kegels creates a synergistic effect, addressing both the physical and psychological aspects of ED.

Tracking Your Progress:

Setting Realistic Goals:

Improving erectile function takes time and dedication. Start by setting realistic and measurable goals, such as completing a specific number of Kegel repetitions daily or noticing incremental improvements in your ability to control pelvic muscles.

Keeping a journal can be helpful. Record your daily exercise routine, dietary habits, stress levels, and any changes in sexual performance. This allows you to track progress over weeks and months, providing motivation and insights into what works best for you.

Recognizing Improvements in Sexual Function:

Improvements may come gradually. Some men notice enhanced control over pelvic muscles within a few weeks, while others may experience stronger erections after a couple of months. Pay attention to subtle changes, such as increased firmness or the ability to sustain an erection longer.

Celebrate milestones, no matter how small. Positive reinforcement boosts motivation and keeps you committed to your routine. If progress stalls, consider consulting a healthcare professional for guidance and support.

By understanding how Kegel exercises work, integrating them with other therapies, and tracking progress effectively, you can take significant strides toward overcoming ED. The journey may require patience and persistence, but the rewards—enhanced confidence, improved relationships, and a healthier life—are well worth the effort.

ENHANCING SEXUAL PERFORMANCE AND CONFIDENCE

Kegel exercises have long been recognized as a powerful tool for improving men's sexual health and overall confidence. This chapter delves into how these exercises can significantly enhance sexual performance, improve stamina, and bolster self-esteem, ultimately contributing to a fulfilling and healthy intimate life.

Improved Blood Flow and Stamina:

The Role of Pelvic Floor Muscles in Sexual Performance:

The pelvic floor muscles play a crucial role in sexual function. These muscles, including the pubococcygeus (PC) muscle, support the bladder, bowel, and sexual organs. When these muscles are strong and well-toned, they can:

I. Enhance blood flow to the genital area, a critical factor for achieving and maintaining erections.

II. Improve control over ejaculation, enabling greater stamina during intimate moments.

III. Heighten sensitivity and pleasure during sexual activity by increasing awareness and strength in the pelvic region.

Regular Kegel exercises can help men gain better control over these muscles, leading to improved performance and endurance in the bedroom.

How Kegel Exercises Improve Stamina:

By targeting the pelvic floor muscles, Kegel exercises can:

1. Strengthen the muscles responsible for erectile function, ensuring better rigidity and sustainability.

2. Increase the duration of sexual activity by delaying ejaculation through enhanced muscular control.

3. Promote recovery after climax, allowing for shorter refractory periods and the potential for greater intimacy.

These benefits make Kegel exercises a simple yet effective way to boost physical stamina and enhance sexual confidence.

Boosting Self-Esteem Through Exercise:

Mental and Emotional Benefits of Physical Fitness:

Beyond physical improvements, Kegel exercises can profoundly impact mental and emotional well-being. Engaging in regular physical fitness activities, including Kegels, offers numerous psychological benefits:

I. Increased Confidence: Knowing that you are taking steps to improve your sexual health can boost self-esteem and self-image.

II. Reduced Anxiety: Better control over sexual performance can alleviate performance-related stress and anxiety.

III. Improved Mood: Physical activity, even as focused as Kegels, releases endorphins, promoting a positive mood and reducing symptoms of depression.

A stronger connection between mind and body, fostered by Kegel exercises, leads to greater confidence not only in intimate settings but in other areas of life as well.

Kegel Exercises for Longevity in Sexual Health:

Sustaining Benefits Over Time:

One of the most compelling advantages of Kegel exercises is their long-term impact on sexual health. Unlike temporary solutions, consistent practice of Kegels provides enduring benefits:

I. Prevention of Age-Related Decline: As men age, the pelvic floor muscles naturally weaken. Regular Kegels can counteract this decline, maintaining sexual performance and overall pelvic health.

I. Support for Prostate Health: Strengthening the pelvic floor muscles may aid in preventing or alleviating symptoms associated with prostate issues, such as urinary incontinence or erectile dysfunction.

II. Continued Confidence: Sustained improvements in sexual stamina and control help men feel assured and capable throughout their lives.

Building a Routine for Lifelong Benefits:

To maximize the longevity of these benefits, consider the following tips:

1. Consistency is Key: Perform Kegel exercises daily, aiming for at least three sets of 10-15 repetitions.

2. Integrate into Daily Activities: Practice Kegels discreetly during routine tasks such as driving, sitting at your desk, or watching TV.

3. Seek Professional Guidance: Consult a healthcare provider or physical therapist specializing in pelvic health to ensure proper technique and progression.

By incorporating Kegel exercises into your daily routine, you can enjoy enhanced sexual performance and confidence well into the future.

Kegel exercises for men have long been celebrated for their role in improving sexual health. However, their benefits extend far beyond the bedroom. In this chapter, we explore the profound impact these exercises can have on bladder and bowel control, core stability, and recovery after surgery. By understanding these advantages, men can appreciate the broader value of incorporating Kegel exercises into their daily routines.

Improved Bladder and Bowel Control:

One of the most significant non-sexual benefits of Kegel exercises is improved bladder and bowel control. These exercises strengthen the pelvic floor muscles, which play a vital role in maintaining continence and preventing conditions that affect urinary and bowel function.

Managing Incontinence:

Urinary incontinence, whether occasional leakage during a sneeze or more frequent accidents, can be a distressing condition. Kegel exercises target the muscles responsible for closing the bladder and urethra, helping men regain control. Regular practice can:

I. Reduce or eliminate stress incontinence caused by pressure on the bladder.

II. Improve urge incontinence by enhancing the bladder's ability to retain urine.

III. Minimize the likelihood of nighttime accidents.

Preventing Prolapse:

While prolapse is more commonly associated with women, men can also experience pelvic organ prolapse, particularly after surgeries like prostatectomy. Kegel exercises help support the pelvic organs, reducing the risk of prolapse and its associated discomfort.

Strengthening Core Stability:

The pelvic floor muscles are a crucial component of the body's core. Alongside the abdominal, back, and diaphragm muscles, they contribute to overall stability and fitness.

How Pelvic Floor Health Impacts Overall Fitness:

A strong pelvic floor improves posture and balance by supporting the lower spine and pelvis. This foundation allows men to perform physical activities with greater efficiency and reduced risk of injury. Benefits include:

I. Enhanced athletic performance through better core engagement.

II. Reduced back pain by alleviating pressure on the lumbar spine.

III. Improved breathing mechanics, as a stable core supports the diaphragm.

Incorporating Kegel exercises into fitness routines can amplify the effects of traditional core workouts, leading to a more resilient and capable body.

Post-Surgery Recovery:

Pelvic surgeries, such as prostate or hernia operations, can weaken the pelvic floor muscles. Kegel exercises are powerful tools for rehabilitation, helping men recover strength and function.

Helping Men Recover from Prostate or Pelvic Surgeries:

After prostate surgery, many men experience urinary incontinence or diminished pelvic function. Kegel exercises can:

I. Accelerate recovery by restoring muscle strength and coordination.

II. Reduce the duration and severity of post-surgical incontinence.

III. Improve quality of life by enhancing confidence in daily activities.

Healthcare providers often recommend beginning Kegel exercises pre-surgery to build a strong foundation and continuing them post-surgery to support recovery.

Beyond their well-known sexual health benefits, Kegel exercises offer a wide array of advantages that can profoundly enhance men's quality of life. From improving bladder and bowel control to strengthening core stability and aiding post-surgery recovery, these exercises are a simple yet powerful tool. By embracing Kegel exercises, men can take proactive steps toward overall well-being and long-term health.

CONCLUSION

In this book, we have explored the importance of strengthening the pelvic floor muscles through Kegel exercises for overcoming erectile dysfunction (ED) and boosting overall sexual function. As we've seen, these simple yet effective exercises can significantly improve blood flow, enhance muscle control, and ultimately restore confidence in sexual health.

The pelvic floor muscles play a crucial role in supporting erectile function, urinary control, and overall sexual well-being. Regularly practicing Kegel exercises can help to strengthen these muscles, leading to long-term benefits such as improved erectile function, heightened sexual pleasure, and a reduction in symptoms of ED. By incorporating these exercises into your daily routine, you are taking a proactive approach toward better health and more fulfilling sexual experiences.

Encouragement to Take the First Step:

Taking the first step toward incorporating Kegel exercises into your daily life can feel daunting, but remember that every journey starts with a single step. Building confidence in your ability to regain control of your pelvic health can make all the difference in overcoming ED and improving your overall quality of life. The benefits you will experience from consistent practice are well worth the effort, so don't hesitate to begin today.

If you need additional guidance or support, several resources are available to help you on your journey. There are numerous apps designed to track your progress and remind you to complete your daily Kegel exercises. You may also find helpful books and professional services, such as pelvic health specialists or sexual health counselors, who can provide personalized advice and support. Don't hesitate to explore these resources to enhance your practice and gain further insights into optimizing your sexual health.

By committing to these exercises and integrating them into your daily routine, you are investing in your future well-being and sexual vitality. Take control of your health and unlock your full potential today!

THE END